The Long Wait
the
Caregiver's
Guide
to Survival

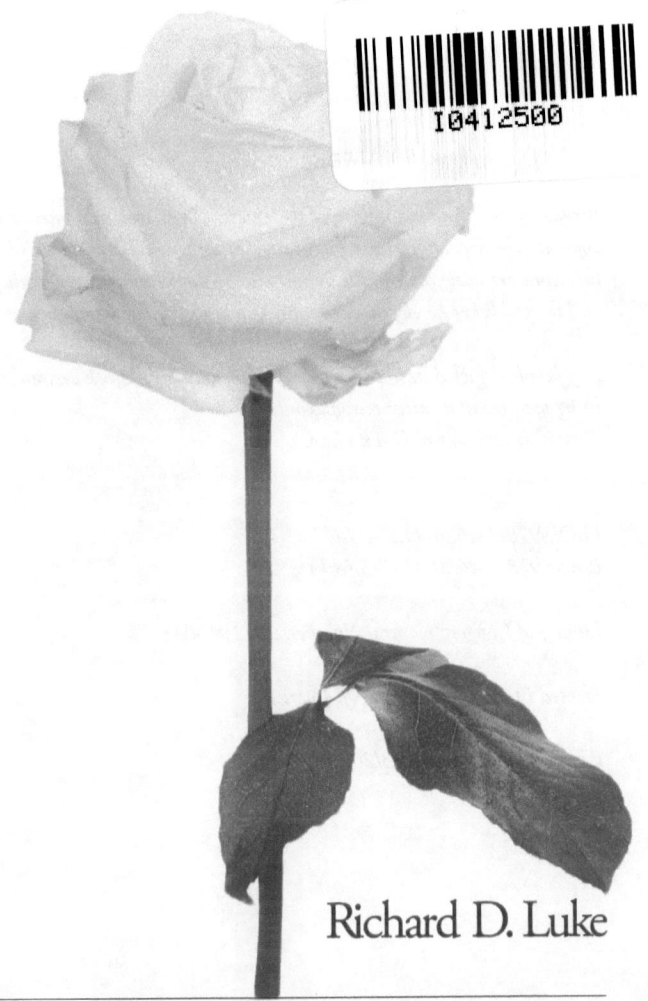

Richard D. Luke

THE LONG WAIT
THE CAREGIVER'S GUIDE TO SURVIVAL

iUniverse books may be ordered through booksellers or by contacting:

iUniverse
1663 Liberty Drive
Bloomington, IN 47403
www.iuniverse.com
1-800-Authors (1-800-288-4677)

ISBN: 978-1-4620-4126-8 (sc)
ISBN: 978-1-4620-4127-5 (ebk)

Library of Congress Control Number: 2011913043

Printed in the United States of America

iUniverse rev. date: 07/23/2011

About The Author

Richard D. Luke has had a varied business career. An artist since the age of 5, he has grown with his talents. After working for 15 years preparing and illustrating management presentations in the Aerospace Industry to be shown to the President, Joint Chiefs of Staff, and the famous rocket scientist, Werner Von Braun, he branched out into another field.

He opened his own Advertising and Commercial Art agency near Los Angeles and continued with his expertise in illustrating and designing creative art for his clients. He is also a Southern California animal portrait artist having been commissioned to do portraits of champion dogs and others in the animal kingdom.

He ventured into the Mortuary and Cemetery field after his mother passed away in 1989. He rose quickly to Division Sales Manager with Rose Hills Memorial Park in Whittier California, the largest in the world with over 3000 acres, and was a formidable player in the overall sales revenue.

Moving to Palm Springs in 1993, he was sales manager for Living Desert and Entertainment on channel 7 and also the Palm Canyon Times. He then became very involved with the western cities in the valley, and was very busily engaged as an Ambassador for each city. Since then, he has turned to his writing talents, having published his first cookbook, and now this book.

Then in 1995, his wife developed Alzheimer's disease. He

went thru the first 4 years of home care while continuing his responsibilities for the cities. It took its toll, raising his stress factor to the power of ten. He placed her in a nursing home where she is now, unable to move, talk, eat, and memory totally gone…and he still tries to help feed her when he can. Thus, the purpose of this book. To enlighten you with facts and warnings that you will face and the problems that will occur that haven't even crossed your mind as you read this.

It is his hope that millions will see what they will be up against with the trials and tribulations that will happen, and will change their lives forever. It is his intention that this book be the key to your survival.

For more information:
luke@creativeartisticproductions.com
www.creativeartisticproductions.com

Preface

By Noreen Bumby, D.O.

The book written by Richard Luke, *The Caregiver's Guide to Survival* of Alzheimer's disease provides an in depth insight into what the family and others are in store for and how to handle situations before they arise. I first met Richard and Wally (his wife and a patient with Alzheimer's disease) during a research study on treatment and pharmacology trials that lasted for 26 weeks. What took place was a long and arduous relationship between the staff and this family. The observation was the commitment of a husband seeking answers to an insurmountable problem of a progressive disease with little to no hope for improvement.

During the treatment process we observed Wally making some adjustments with little improvement based on the pharmacology treatment plan. What Richard was able to do was develop his own plan of action on taking care of their personal business and increasing duties of a caregiver. The heart breaking knowledge was that his partner in life was not going to be able to enjoy retirement and their future together as a couple was ending.

Regarding research, there are multiple avenues of research being developed from surgical interventions to vaccines, hormones, and other newer protocols are being explored all the time. There have been advancements made in pharmacological treatment that helps with the memory, however showing only short term progress. We in the field of research are hopeful that as the population ages the advancement in discovering a long lasting treatment will be provided to those who suffer from Alzheimer's disease.

Until such treatments are available, it is important that the caregiver receives support, guidance and assistance in their role as a caregiver. This book is an absolute must read for anyone who is taking care of a loved one, friend or relative who has the diagnosis of Alzheimer's disease.

Noreen Bumby, D.O.
Gero-Psychiatrist
Investigator at the Southwest Institute for Clinical Research

Dedication

This book is dedicated to my wife Wally and to every other family whose lives have just been altered by bringing stress, fear and intrepidation into their lives. To give hope for those caught in this web of unfortunate fate. To give courage where there is fear. To give insight and advice on decisions to one who has been snagged into this web of despair. I have managed to come through the first 13 years of seeing my loved one fade away. Time will be a key player as well as your status in life, and how you are going to survive the test of that time, which will be spent just holding on to your own existence.

It is intended to intelligently convey the message of love and responsibility that a caregiver is going to have to muster to absorb the violence, the inability to converse, or to understand the language of love that you are mutually re-expressing. If one does not, then the caregiver may fall prey to the sobering statistic that 65% of all 24/7 caregivers will die before the death of the one they are caring for, because of the stress they will endure. This is a fact.

What you must do, what you must prepare for...alas, it will be...

A LONG WAIT.

Contents

The Long Wait
the
Caregiver's
Guide
to Survival

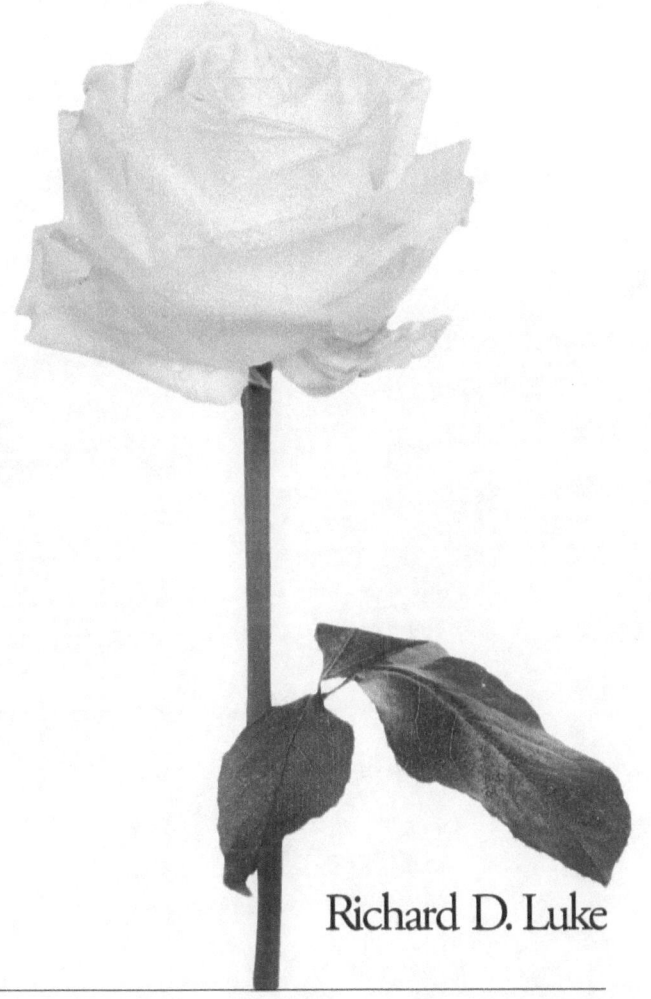

Richard D. Luke

Chapter 1

In The Beginning...

Yes, you're right...it's the first 10 words of the Bible. In the beginning, God created the Heaven and the Earth. Why should we mention that? Well, because that's where everything started.

Not only was "good" put upon the Earth but "bad" was also. Now you can take the word "bad" and apply it to almost everything that goes wrong in our lives - personal, or in business, or in the countries of the world. We have been fighting insurrections, wars, tragedies, illness, starvation, and human sacrifice - all bad. But then comes the human evaluation that touches our lives, each and every one of us. And in this case....illnesses.

There are illnesses that preempt the need for a cure. Illnesses that may not take the "cure" and illnesses that will need the curing salvation of all that medicine has to offer for a long time...and no guarantee for success.

Then there are the illnesses for which there is no cure, and that is where we are in this book and revelation to all who come under that title and the caregivers who have been given the unwanted, and daunting task of being the only venue to which the ill have a chance of accepting that which they are being dealt with in their lives. Age? Nope, doesn't compute. Why? Because illnesses can strike at any age. Oh sure, there are medicines that can delay, or comfort an illness but don't cure it, if you live through the side effects of many of the medicines today that promise you total submission of the disease…as long as you put up with the side effects or even death when taking many of the prescriptions today that are offered.

Today we are on the brink of new treatments using the latest in discoveries of such findings as stem cells. They are just coming into the research scene now with the availability of their use in some states. It won't be long when that will be the normal practice. The stem cells alone will be promising in the treatment of Parkinson's, Lou Gehrig's disease, spinal column disorders , and of course the cursor of them all - ALZHEIMER'S DISEASE, the focus of this book.

There are a number of prescription medicines out there now that are being utilized for this disease, but….the side affects, and most of all, you really cannot tell if they are working or not. There are alternative claims as well and vitamins or herbs that make their name known. Once Vitamin E was mentioned to prolong the disease…then it was discounted that it did not produce the wanted effects. Aricept is the leading drug… however it comes in 5 mg and 10 mg. I have not seen much difference…whether it was helping or not. Yes, studies are going on, but they are not much closer to the cause and cure as before. All they can claim is that they "may" help - but surely not cure. They just drag out the inevitable.

Well, let's play the role out. It was one evening when we were taking the dog for a walk. Wally (my beloved wife) asked… what month is this…she said October….it was June. I knew then something was happening. So, as the months progressed, I noticed she was repeating what she just said…and asking the same questions as I just answered. It became monitored as I saw it happening time and time again. Then, washing dishes, I washed, she dried…"Where does this go?" was the phrase that struck the hardest for me. I knew then that it was time for an examination. Now, you know what is going to happen…you are trying your best now to make her/him comfortable…but… you haven't seen anything yet. Pretty soon YOU will have to be comforted for the tide is about to change. Okay, now let's get to the examination.

Make your appointment…..that done? Good. Now you must be in the room with her…don't let the doctor keep you out… you must know everything from this point forward. The first thing the doctor will do is of course, hear the heart, take the vitals, all those steps first so that he is sure he will get paid for it. Then he will hand your loved one a paper with 7 questions. That's right, only 7. A real test isn't it …hmmm, well, I would have trouble doing what they expect myself, but, let's move on. Questions asking name, address, what day it is, etcetera, then the fun begins. He will mention three things of object. Then he will wait 5 minutes, and then ask your loved one to repeat what he just mentioned.

Then he will start with 100 and ask your loved one to count backwards. After 10 minutes of that little gem, He will probably tell you that there is an indication of Dementia which 90% fall into the Alzheimer's category. Now you are advised to get a second opinion…AND YOU SHOULD. And the next doctor will do the same thing. If he comes with the same conclusion, he will tell you and report back to your first doctor.

THEN THE FIRST DOCTOR IS ORDERED BY LAW TO SEND IN THE NOTICE TO THE DEPARTMENT OF MOTOR VEHICLES TO TAKE AWAY THEIR DRIVER'S LICENSE. That is where the fun begins for your loved one - either their need for the car for work or to just travel from day to day. Now your loved one will start the downhill slide, for he/she, in their own eyes, has lost their independence.

You can't wait to start taking action to protect them, your home, the rest of the family, and yourself, for from this instant on, you are in danger as well. More on that later. The shock wave has started and as it moves about your brain you think "Oh, I can handle this." Well, my unsuspecting friend, stronger people than you have fallen and lay prone on the ground as the Paramedics work feverishly and unsuccessfully to save you. The stress on your system will be so bazaar that you will want to cry out and your strength will diminish. You are about to enter into a lifestyle so different from what you are now enjoying, that the accumulated chores and responsibilities will change what you are doing and you will have to face making choices, for now the game has changed and the priorities have changed with it for your day to day activities.

Yes, my friend, now listen carefully, for you will see a difference in your loved one that may astonish you and shock you, and wear you down to a frizzle…and if you think that it won't happen…then just the emotions of it all may kill you…

and I am serious about that.

Now granted, there are other diseases - Parkinson's, Lou
Gehrig's disease, Spinal Chord Abnormalities, and others
that play with the same deck of cards for the caregivers. And
yes, now that you have been told that your loved one has
been diagnosed with Alzheimer's you may see some shaking
moments in the beginning and make an appointment to see a
Parkinson's specialist for it can run parallel with the disease. It
can confuse you for shaking alone does not necessarily mean
Parkinson's; other physical tests in the doctor's office will
confirm one way or another. But don't go rushing off scared
as a rabbit...look for those signs. Get on the internet; learn of
the latest findings on both diseases. I did. You see, Alzheimer's
disease cannot really be officially diagnosed until an autopsy
has been performed, but the doctors can give a well educated
guess based on their findings.

I even corresponded with the Alzheimer's research laboratory
in Dublin Ireland and spoke with the head scientist there. They
came out with a supposed vaccine, but in Minnesota they found
40 cases of Hepatitis B and stopped the production. But I do
have evidence of a lab in Phoenix, Arizona that did use it and
reversed the symptoms...then the vaccine was pulled from the
market. I understand they are going to try again. Time will tell.

Time, it has no meaning now. Day, night, afternoon, morning,
it all will require additional physical equipment, construction,
and day to day routine changes...like I said, you have just
started. And, the main question all will ask...WHAT DO I DO

NOW? Your heart has just plunged to the depths of your soul in complete anguish for you are lost in a sea of indeterminate decisions and where do you go, how will I handle this, I have no money, I have a job, I cant stay home, I cant afford a resident nurse...again you repeat..."WHAT DO I DO NOW?"

Now you have to read on because you are now spellbound by learning of what is to be and you are going to need all the help you can get from family, friends, neighbors, the Police Department, the Fire Department....and again, this is just the beginning.

Chapter 2

What is Alzheimer's Disease?
An educated discussion of what is known.

The first breath that comes from your mouth as the doctor finishes his findings and you are sitting confounded is: "What is Alzheimer's disease?" The doctor looks at you and winces as he is about to bring the world down around you.

There are now more than 5 million people in the United Sates living with Alzheimer's disease. This number includes 4.9 million people over the age of 65 and between 200,000 and 500,000 people under age 65 with early-onset Alzheimer's disease and other dementias.

When Dr. Alzheimer in about 1914 discovered the link between the normal and abnormal functions of the memory process and made it known, it was generally not accepted and was tabled by the scientific community. In the 1940's people with memory problems were labeled as senile and placed into an institution or reasonable facsimile and visited by the family when possible. Well it was not until 1986 that it was brought to light again and was researched extensively. Then it was labeled as Alzheimer's disease after its founder. But at that time much was still to be tested and known about the problem because many were coming down with it and all those who in the past that were diagnosed differently. Again, I repeat, you cannot diagnose Alzheimer's disease officially until an autopsy has been performed once the person as expired. So, with the

introductory testing that is given, a very close perception
is given and to its relationship to Dementia. Yes, an MRI is
necessary to view the brain and its relative space between the
scull because the degree of separation is important.

Alzheimer's disease is a progressive brain disorder that
gradually destroys a person's memory and ability to learn,
reason, make judgments, communicate and carry out daily
activities. As Alzheimer's progresses, individuals may also
experience changes in personality and behavior, such as
anxiety, suspiciousness or agitation, as well as delusions or
hallucinations.

Alzheimer's is the most common form of dementia, a group
of conditions that all gradually destroy brain cells and lead to
progressive decline in mental functions. Vascular dementia,
another common form, results from reduced blood flow to
the brain's nerve cells. In some cases, Alzheimer's disease
and vascular dementia can occur together in a condition
called "mixed dementia." Other causes of dementia include
frontotemporal dementia, dementia with Lewy bodies,
Creutzfeldt-Jakob disease and Parkinson's disease.

Alzheimer's disease advances at widely different rates. People
with Alzheimer's die an average of four to six years after
determination, but the cells that control memory and thinking
skills are affected first, but as the disease progresses, cells die
in other regions of the brain. The duration of the disease can
vary from three to twenty years, the averaging being around 8
years.

Eventually, the person with Alzheimer's will need complete care. If the individual has no other serious illness, the loss of brain function itself will cause death. Other organs such as the liver, kidneys, and heart will be impaired with the heart muscle the last to show complications and malfunction.

"Early-stage" is the early part of Alzheimer's disease when problems with memory, thinking and concentration may begin to appear in a doctor's interview or medical tests. Individuals in the early-stage typically need minimal assistance with simple daily routines. At the time of a determination of the disease, with the individual not necessarily in the early stage of the disease: he or she may have progressed beyond the early stage.

Alzheimer's disease leads to nerve cell death and tissue loss throughout the brain. Over time, the brain shrinks dramatically, affecting nearly all its functions. Plaques, abnormal clusters of protein fragments, build up between the nerve cells. Dead and dying nerve cells contain tangles, which are made up of twisted strands of another protein. Scientists are still not sure what causes cell death and tissue in the Alzheimer brain, but plaques and tangles are prime suspects.

Plaques form when protein pieces called Beta-Amyloid clump together. Beta-Amyloid comes from a larger protein found in the fatty membrane surrounding nerve cells. Beta-Amyloid is chemically sticky and gradually builds up into plaques.

Signals traveling through the neuron forest form the basis of memories, thoughts, and feelings. Neurons are the main type of cells destroyed by Alzheimer's disease.

Alzheimer's disease disrupts both the way electrical charges travel within the cells and the activity of neurotransmitters.

Specific Activity patterns change throughout life as we meet new people, have new experiences and acquire new skills. The patterns also change when Alzheimer's disease, or a related disorder, disrupts nerve cells and their connection to one another.

Tangles destroy a vital cell transport system mode of proteins. The transport system is organized in orderly parallel strands somewhat like rail road tracks. Food molecules, cell parts, and other key materials travel along the "tracks" operation called "Tau" which helps the tracks stay straight. In areas where tangles are forming, Tau collapses into twisted strands called tangles. The tracks can no longer stay straight. They fall apart and disintegrate. Nutrients and other essential supplies can no longer move through the cells which eventually die.

Plaques and tangles tend to spread through the cortex in a predictable pattern as Alzheimer's disease progresses. The rate of progression varies greatly. People with AD (Alzheimer's disease) live an average of 8 years but some people may survive up to 20 years.

The course of the disease depends in part on age at diagnosis and whether a person has other health conditions.

Earlier Alzheimer's

Changes may begin 20 years or more before diagnosis. Plaques and tangles can be detected and begin to form in these areas: learning, memory, thinking and planning.

Mild to Moderate:

Individuals generally last 2-10 years. More plaques and tangles in memory and thinking. Has trouble handling money, expressing oneself and organizing thoughts. Recognizes friends and family.

Severe Alzheimer's disease:

May last 1-8 years. Most of cortex is seriously damaged. Lost ability to communicate, caring for self and recognizing family.

Currently there are 5.5 million in the U.S. over 65, and 500,000 under 65 affected with Alzheimer's disease.

THE WARNING SIGNS OF ALZHEIMERS

There is the natural process of memory loss as we get older. Forgetting where you put your key is one thing …but forgetting what they are used for is a possible sign that there could be something more than what is on the surface. However, the symptoms of Alzheimer's disease reach far further than just lapses of memory.

People that are experiencing the ravages of Alzheimer's disease find that simple communication, learning, thinking, and reasoning is invading their ability to comprehend simple tasks, work, social activities, and family life.

There is no clear-cut line between normal changes and warning signs. One must look for those odd moments that cause you to question their reasoning. So, here are the 10 warning signs that may or may not preclude that your loved one may have a problem, and you need to deal with it as soon as possible.

1. Memory Loss:
Forgetting recently learned information is one of the most common early sign of dementia. A person begins to forget more often and is unable to recall the information later.

What is normal?
Forgetting names of appointments occasionally.

2. Difficultly performing familiar tasks:
People with Alzheimer's often find it hard to plan or complete everyday tasks. Individuals may lose the concentration to prepare a meal, making a telephone call or playing a game.

What is normal?
Occasionally forgetting who came into the room or what you planned to say to another person.

3. Problems with a language:
Those afflicted with AD (Alzheimer's disease) often forget simple words or substitute unusual words, making their speech or writing hard to understand. For example: they may not be able to bring up the word for the hood of a car…and say instead "the thing that covers the engine".

What is normal?
Occasionally having trouble finding the right word.

4. Disorientation to time and place:

This warning sign is probably the most important one because
it really takes danger to the highest level. One can get lost in
their own neighborhood and can't find their way back home.
Or, worst yet, if they are driving...they forget the rules of the
road or which way to turn...and that's why as soon as one
finds out the sad news, the law requires the doctor to send a
letter to the department of Motor Vehicles informing them
that your loved one has been "diagnosed" with AD. The state
will pull their license (California anyway). They cannot drive
anymore...and that is devastating to your loved one.

What is normal?
Forgetting what day is or where you were intending to go.
How many times have you entered a room and said to yourself,
"now, what was I supposed to get in here?"

5. Poor or decreased judgment:

This is a sign that may promote your concern. Let's say it
is 100 degrees outside and your loved one has just put on a
sweater of jacket to go outside...that doesn't take much to ask
a question...you may not get the answer its 50 degrees outside
and they have just a pair of shorts on and a T-shirt or blouse.
Now you need to take note. Maybe they are doing a recipe and
have done it a dozen times, their favorite and yours also. But,
they have forgotten the recipe or they put in 4 eggs instead
of two...or bake it at 250 degrees and not at 400 degrees. It's

these things you will have to be alerted to, and watch out for. It's beginning to happen…..and this is just the beginning.

What is normal?
Making a questionable or debatable decision from time to time.

6. Problems with abstract thinking:

Someone with AD may have unusual difficulty performing complex mental tasks, like forgetting what numbers are for and how they should be used. That's why crossword puzzles, number games, monopoly, or other games using numbers is helpful. And again, you say…. I don't have the time…I have to work…now what? You are beginning to see the need of a daytime location for you loved one. Yes, they do exist. They are day care centers that you pay a fee for the day, and they are cared for, fed, and engage in activities, games, crafts, etc. I had one for my wife and it was nice, but she was passed the point of understanding the instructions and the efforts were rather null and void. They are helpful, but there comes a time of diminishing return and you may need to start looking for a more permanent facility. DON'T EVEN THINK YOU CAN DO IT YOURSELF AND KEEP YOUR SANITY….YOU CAN'T.

What is normal?
Finding it challenging to balance a checkbook? Sure, been there, done that. But let them do it to see if and when, and where they begin to almost stop in the process.

7. Misplacing things.

Oh boy, this is where the fun begins. You open the refrigerator and find her set of earrings or maybe the dust rag or box of soap. Now this is where you step in and start doing the dishes, if you are not already doing that chore, and putting the dishes in the proper cupboards because your loved one will place them in the wrong cupboard and you will be frustrated and your blood pressure begins to rise. A person with AD may put things in unusual places, for example, an iron in the freezer, a wristwatch in the sugar bowl…see what I mean?

What is normal?

Misplacing keys or a wallet temporarily. Now let me repeat… forgetting where you put your keys is one thing…forgetting what they are for (house) is a concern.

8. Changes in mood or behavior.

Someone with AD may show rapid mood swings – from calm to tears to anger – for no apparent reason you can see. Now, you have to watch this carefully. The anger can appear and can be very serious, even violent, and dangerous for you. They may pick up a lamp and throw it at you. They may be mad for no reason at all. You must protect yourself - a knife in the chest or a skillet over the head doesn't feel good. Now I don't mean this is going to happen in all cases of AD…but violence has, and to what degree will it explode. My wife did for about a week, but only aggravation and short temper and conversation…I was lucky.

What is normal?
Occasionally feeling sad or moody.

9. Changes in personality?

The personalities of people with AD can change dramatically.
They may become extremely confused, suspicious, fearful or
outwardly dependent on a family member. The point of being
suspicious or confused is very likely. The confusion is most
prominent. Or, they may draw back and not say very much at
all…period. They are losing touch with reality. If they spoke
a foreign language, they may even revert to it and forget
English…but in my case she forgot her German and spoke
only her good English. She couldn't translate documents or
remember pictures of the family or who they were…so get
those wanted pictures done now with names on the family
members. I didn't get all that, and now I don't remember who
some of her relatives were. No names.

What is normal?
People's personalities do change somewhat with age. That's
why it is important to mingle with others, play card games, or
go out into the public to meet new people - anything to keep
them thinking and the mind active.

10. Loss of appetite:

A person with AD may become very passive, sitting in front
of the TV for hours, sleeping more than usual or not wanting
to do usual activities. I didn't have that problem….she worked
constantly around the house after her retirement, so I didn't
notice it, and besides, I could still go to work at that time.

What is normal?
Sometimes feeling weary of work or social obligations.

Here is the difference between AD and normal age-related memory changes.

With AD memory change	Normal age-related
Forgets entire experiences	Forgets part of an experience
Rarely remembers later	Often remembers later
Is gradually unable to follow written/spoken directions	Is usually able to use notes as reminders
Is gradually unable to care for self	Is usually able to care for self

Chapter 3

The Change In Our Daily Routines

Sometimes in our normal conversations during the day, we once in a while forget that we just asked a question …and our mind wandered for a moment as we got involved with something and then ask it again…that's not a problem. It's when your loved one asks what day it is…and 5 minutes later asks it again or maybe again another 5 minutes after that.

THIS IS THE BEGINNING. This is where you must realize that there is a problem. And what do you say to your loved one after that? That's right…you tell her in an increasing tone of voice, "you asked me that!" Think it won't happen? ...oh yes it will, over and over again. That is the first test of your ability to withhold your frustration, but it too will falter and you will find that out as the condition worsens.

You are going to hate those words for you are going to repeat them a thousand times over as your loved one now switches to other statements that will confuse you and start to have its affect on your mental stability. Oh, it could be, what time is it, or to ask you if you need a drink of water… again …and again…. Or just a sentence of the agenda maybe for the day…I have to go to the store…I have to go to the store…I have…you see what I mean? You will have to answer back because they DO NOT KNOW THEY JUST SAID IT OR ASKED IT. Now, this is one of the FIRST signs of trouble. As in the last chapter about what to do if you see those signs and head for your doctor and a second testing by another doctor.

One of the hardest things you will encounter along this line is the everyday chores one does around the house - simple everyday chores that do not require much thought or action, just routine. Sure, but those routines are going to cause you to make decisions and changes in your life to where you will begin to show anger…the pitfall of being a caregiver. Oh, you say you don't get angry or upset…after all, it's your loved one.

Wrong! You will, trust me. Oh, I don't mean violent anger, just complete aggravation and impatience with what is happening.

I started to see the changes in her right then, and in myself. I had many responsibilities to take care of in my business and my civic functions. And telling her that she just said that will start another of the angers…only with your loved one. Wally would tell me, "Don't tell me that, I just forgot!" Then 5 minutes later…say the same thing again…and I then learned after much of the wrangling and outbursts, to let it go…and that is going to be the hardest task you will start with…notice I didn't say, "that you will have" because as I said in the last chapter…THIS IS JUST THE BEGINNING.

To repeat, I think the very first time I noticed a change was when we went for our nightly walk, and she asked "what month is this October?" No, I replied, it's June. I knew then that it was changing. Her brother and wife visited several times from Germany and had gone through the same predicament with Wally's half Aunt. She started to lose it fast and the legality with all of it was overwhelming for the family and a caregiver was assigned from a friend there in Florida. The amount of legal help stacked up with papers, court documents declaring her incapacitated, and results of those court hearings were coming in monthly. At this time, Wally did not have any signs and we were saying, "gee, what a shame" for she loved her aunt and Uncle. They helped the family out of harms way after their home was bombed during the Hamburg Germany blitz from Great Britain. Yes it has been said that the concussion of the bombs could have had a part in the cells being jarred or the plaque increasing and causing separation from the scull. It is just a theory. Her aunt had to sell the home, furnishings, etc., and was placed into an assisted living facility. More on that later because your eyes are going to pop out when you will hear about those facilities compared to nursing homes. Finally Wally's Aunt passed away but not for another couple years or so. All the monies were depleted…how? You ask… well that's for another chapter along with the facilities.

At this point in time when we took a walk that night, I began to fear what her behavior was to be. Her brother and his wife were here and began to notice the repetition of phrases and questions. I said it was now time to go for the examination.

We made the appointment. The doctor chose the test of 7 questions. There are other tests but the basics are done in this test to determine the longevity of memory retention. He asked the questions and she answered fairly well. Following was the 5 things to remember test. The doctor came back to the 5 things and asked her to repeat them…and she couldn't.

The doctor then suggested a second opinion. We did just that and the results were the same. The doctor had to do what is required by law as I said in the previous chapter. He had to send in the paper to Sacramento that she had been diagnosed with early Alzheimer's disease, and that her California Drivers License would now be revoked and she would not be able to drive.

Can you imagine what that did to her? That took away her independence. That was a shock to her system and mental stability for now she could not drive and do things on her own and she really enjoyed driving and was a good driver. Now you ask, "Why take it away?" Well, because she may be driving and not remember how to get back home…or turn right when she should have turned left. You see how dangerous that could be.

There came another blow to her daily routine and soon to affect mine. We went to the Department of Motor Vehicles and got an identification license. It showed her picture and the normal information. I pondered at what this was going to do to our life and how was I to handle it or even "know" how to handle it. It was a quiet drive home.

As I began to notice the various changes, one occurred which I was in question about. You see, there is another disease that can accompany AD (the short abbreviation used) and that is Parkinson's disease. Why? Because her hand started to shake a little and I had heard that it could be, speaking from those who went through the same thing already. By the way, staying close to "others" are going to be a blessing for you. They will give you strength. Not hope…for there is nothing to hope for…it is a terminal disease.

An appointment was made to see a Parkinson's disease Specialist. He gave a few normal tests…like touch your nose; follow the little light, things like that. He gave her a clean bill that she did not have the disease. And for those of you who are caregivers to one having that disease, it's all the same and this book is focused on all who are caregivers.

It was at least a relief in a way. But it was something to be thankful for it would have been even more debilitating. I was beginning to feel the pressure building within me and I was completely at a loss of what to do next. Life had been good and bad for our family: financial complications, loss of jobs, and the economy. There were pressures of raising a family without engaging in long conversations in their early years so as not to confound them and make it any worse for them. But every family goes through something that tests their endurance but you must learn to be a survivor and we taught our children that principle. Wally had been a real survivor during the war and I had survived being a latch key child with a loving mother who was going through alcoholism. But on the bright side, my last major vacation, before the onset of AD, was one that provided considerable income, enabling me to provide her the best life could offer. She had brought us through tough times and now it was my turn to give her freedom from despair and work and give her the good life she deserved.

Now what, I asked myself. We had not planned for this to

happen, it just did and life throws us those curves to see how strong you really are. It doesn't matter what spiritual beliefs you have, but it helps to have something to turn to for help and self composure. Other changes soon began to surface. We never said that one chore around the house belonged to either of us or our children…it was a family and families share those responsibilities. Wally and I together cooked or washed the dishes. It didn't matter who did what, it was get it done. Well, that was to change. With the children now grown, married and living their lives, we decided to move to our retirement site and a new life. After five years that "new life" changed abruptly. She would take immeasurable time washing now and maybe re-washing something. So, I took over washing the dishes. Now the next change began to take place. "WHERE DOES THIS GO?" It sounds like a simple question except it was dinner plates and it went where it had always been placed, in the cupboard. Ah yes….but which one you say. I answered her with "here or there". But then it became a multiple repeat of the "where" and it was then you realized you will have to make another change in your daily routine.

The answer is, place little identifying signs on all the cupboards revealing what is in each of the cupboards. Hmmm, well, that wouldn't look very nice so I decided not to and to mainly take over both wash and dry. Our dishwasher wasn't working anyway. But that did not stop the constant questioning of where something was in the cupboards. Now that didn't mean that it was constant in the way that it was all the time. You see, it doesn't work that way. The mind can move in and out of reality. One day may be completely different than the day before. She may well have remembered for that day or a period during the day. That is the way AD changes from day to day activities.

 It won't stop there. Maybe you have thought of it by now… and you asked yourself…what about the cooking? BINGO! You hit it on the nose. She loved to cook as I did. Our hope was to publish a cookbook together with recipes from all over the world and our families and our own creation. More on that later. What about cooking? Simple. What if she turns on the gas….AND FORGETS SHE HAS IT ON. Well we have all done that and that's not a problem for it to happen once in a great while. But, to have it happen with AD, you can see where I am going with this. FIRE…or a burned meal. Not intentional, but the mind gave away in that she has something on the stove. I don't need to go into details on a train wreck waiting to happen. Yes, you are correct, I started to take over the cooking. I could have her do other things, but I handled the stove.

Now I have added chief cook and bottle washer to MY daily routine. You could test her once in a while to see if she was on track that day. I tried to start giving her the challenges. You see, she now knows that she has the disease and knows what the outcome will be, remembering her Aunt in Florida. She knows that every little change in her mental jogging means a tougher road ahead. And it irritates her no end. Well, we have the washing, drying, putting away, and cooking out of the way. You may think that if you will, but again, this is just the beginning.

Sure it's routine to just sit down at a table and start eating. Not to one who has AD. I began to see changes occurring. I would put the food on the plate and she may sit starring at it a while before picking up a fork or spoon. So I would have to begin guiding her and showing her the process the fork should take to pick up the food. You see, now you have to wonder that she is deciding what a fork or spoon is for anyway.

Where this is going now is that if I had a civic function at night, I would now have to start canceling it, for my first call is to Wally. I must now start to sacrifice some of my daily routines so to speak. There goes the pressure building again in my own head. But I knew even at that point and juncture in time that I was going to have to be organized and complete in what I do each day and for her to still function and do laundry etc…there is a long, long way to go.

Well, now it seemed that with the trouble she is having in picking up a fork…the added chore is now in full view, I must now begin feeding her. And that is a challenge. For you see, she is starting to slow down with her chewing. The same food in her mouth may require 5 minutes to eat and swallow. Now in doing this you may see another change…she is holding the food in her mouth. So you have to stroke the throat to excite the throat muscle to come to the forefront and let the food go down her throat. Ooops, hold on…she just bit down on the spoon and you can't get it out…ah yes…the next phase is taking place. Also, Wally has still not swallowed the food. Now what do you do? You can't jerk out the spoon so you must wait…and you will have to call and cancel your meeting you had scheduled. Like I said, this is just the beginning.

Now consider the taking of pills. You are used to taking your vitamins in the morning. However now having your loved one take pills is not like it was before. I would place them out and then give them to her one by one, or at this juncture, she could do it herself. But, soon that will subside. The bottom line is that she would squirrel them in her cheek and not swallow… you have to be aware that this will happen again when you see it happening the first time. Lots of water …and like the food… stroke the throat.

At this point Wally was still moving and walking…hmmm walking…that's another sign of things to happen and your life to change. In her case, she began finding it hard to walk. She had tendonitis in the right foot. So, off to the doctor and a foot and leg brace for several weeks helped, but didn't stop the problem. The daily routine of just walking was coming to an end. Does this happen to all? No, I dare say, but it will become impaired as the cells are destroyed by the plaque that controls the motor movements.

What is happening here is that the normal routines of the day are going to be increasingly difficult for her to manipulate. Washing her teeth, washing, setting, combing her hair add a couple more challenges for your loved one. You are going to see the changes occur right in front of you and you will have to be there to protect your loved one incase she puts herself in harms way. Dressing herself, tying her shoes, putting objects away….into the wrong place.

Let's imagine you have just finished breakfast. Both of you are helping with the clean up and taking care of the dishes, and then you both begin putting things in the refrigerator. You do some…and she does some also…and you are not watching. From now on… watch.

Why? Because they just put their cup of coffee into the refrigerator, including the knife, fork, and spoon. Yes, that's right, now the actions where many things are being placed in odd places…you may even find that cup of coffee in the broom closet. The mind is beginning to work against them now. The recent history memory banks are beginning to shut down. Now the real tasks are working against them. The long term memory will stay strong, but the short term memory is the one to go first. They can remember years ago. Now they have trouble remembering what they had for breakfast. Short term memory tightening up and if you need info for any reason…do it now or lose it. If you have need of historical information, personal history bio, identifying pictures of family, they all need to be addressed and marked. For soon, the long term memory will begin to subside as well, and this is just the beginning.

I remember that we had some very important genealogical documents that need translation for they had to do with WWII and her father's incarceration with the British Army. He was an accountant and on the board of directors of the largest insurance company in Europe, and they figured he must know something of where the gold was hidden. And this was after the ending of the War. He didn't know although his expertise was sought after to re-build much of the infrastructure and financing same. But just wanted some words done, especially on the pictures…aunts, uncles, member of her family…but alas…

didn't happen. I have pictures but no names. Then you must have family pictures as well, and now is the time to go through them and learn who is who, for once your loved one is gone… those names are gone also.

Well, let's change clothes a few times a day…and then the incontinence factor (see chapter 4). You will see changes that transform your loved one into someone you don't know…trust me…and they will not know you. These are the sad facts. You may find her makeup in the refrigerator, or the oven…and what about your sex life…oh…I hit a button didn't I? Well, that will change also. Their mind will soon not be focused, and absence of desire or loving gestures will change. It's not their fault…its just that it may or may not make a difference in yours or their daily routine.

You see, some behavioral actions may occur with one person but not another. An action or behavior that may manifest itself is just plain anger, and they don't know it. Now Wally really never got radical or mean. Just one week of temperament… and I think that was when she was mad at me for reminding her that she had just repeated herself. Remember what I said before, sometimes AD patients have actually been dangerous and threatening.

It has been documented that one has thrown lamps or other objects around the house or became violently wild and threatening. This does not happen routinely. It is the make-up of each individually and each will display their on anger in their own way. Now…what do you do? You may see violent attacks against you…they may throw things at you, or worse with a lethal weapon….You will have to deal with it on each individual basis…and above all… protect yourself. This is just the beginning.

Chapter 4

Incontinence - The Faucet Leaks

As the progression of this dreaded nightmare rolls on, there will come a time when you notice they are washing more underwear. I was doing the wash one day and saw 8 or 10 panties. I thought, why did she use so many in the last two days? Then the unspoken word leaped out at me…she is beginning to lose control of her bladder. Could the bowels be next…what do I do now? Well, I will tell you. You move with the flow of things happening and you start washing more panties. It became evident now that you will need to buy some panty liners to absorb "leaks". For men, there are also liner pads.

At one juncture in time I washed as many as 25 panties in one day. I would mention it to her and it would anger her and "that's the way it is" would be her answer. But it became even worse for the caring phase you are now entering. This is another plaque related failure of brain cells connected to different parts of the body where there is such action such as urinating. It starts off slowly and then increases as I have mentioned. I started using the liner pads …which then also became the thicker ones…and then finally as you will see…you have to switch to adult diapering. And don't forget the odors you will endure.

Now you will enter the arena of no return. Diapering will be the call of the day. And you have to go to work….oh, you are going to have someone come in …I see…at $25 an hour for assistance…not 24 hr…just assistance during the day….forget it….you cant afford it...Let's see 10 hrs a day…because you are not home yet from work…times $25 an hour comes to $1,250.00 a 5-day week or $5,412.50 a month or $64,950.00 a year…Now do you see why families get wiped out? It's easy. So who is going to do it? YOU ARE, MY FRIEND. So now you have to figure if you get family members in…or maybe put your loved one in an assisted living facility…forget that too unless you are well heeled. That could cost you $6,500.00 a month. More on this later. Are you getting my point? You are in deep doo-doo. So, back to the diapers…what a segway… but that has to be a venue you have to explore right then. After your decision to do put your loved one in a facility…then we go there…in a later chapter.

Okay. So now you are facing the diapering phase of all this… Now what? Well, you will have to put it in your budget… yep…$10 a throw for a package of diapers...but what size? You can figure that out okay. If it fits wear it…if not…wear it anyway until you purchase the next size.

You will learn how to put them on IF they cannot do it themselves. Why do I say that? Because, by this time they may not be walking very well, and may have to use a cane, or a tripod cane, or a walker…and can't do it…great if they can. Let's say they cannot. So you have the honor of diapering your loved one. However, there is just one thing…they are incontinent, and there is the morning, afternoon, and evening… hopefully, that's all. You see, my friend, if they can't, and listen

to me…if they can not do it themselves…you are elected.
If you have to work, how can you do it and stay sane? Or
keep from being fired… after all, now you need more money
because of the diaper cost. Hmmm, do you have insurance that
will pay for the diapers? Better check it out…SCAN insurance
does and when I found out they did I implored them to do so
and that saved great sums of money right there. They started
providing the different kinds of diapers needed. What…you
say …how many kinds are there? Oh, a lot…you have light,
medium, heavy, and extra heavy to absorb the flow of urine…
or bowel movement…uhhh I didn't mention that yet did I?
Okay so now you are developing a routine by now…and
getting up at 4 AM to do the bathing of your loved one and then
getting yourself ready to go to work…

Now all this is predicated on whether you can even go to work.
If your loved one can stay home alone and is not fully engulfed
with AD, then you may make it…BUT…if they "walk" and
you are not home…you could be held accountable for elder
abuse…think I am kidding? Hardly!

Because they left the confines of your home and wandered
off somewhere, and you didn't know about it …tch, tch. You
could be fined and/or jailed if that need be. Well, let's pretend
that they are okay. If they can in the beginning function
themselves…that's great. BUT if not, then you are going to be
called to the helm faster than you could realize.

So, now the day is over. The evening has fallen. You are now
cooking the dinner, oh yes, you took over that job when your

loved one left the fire on the stove and set a towel on fire…
yep. Dinner over…you watch a little TV and now it's time for
beddy bye. They help you get ready of course, if they can walk
into the bathroom…otherwise it's your call. So you put on a
diaper …no, no, no, you put on two diapers…to protect during
the night. And kiss goodnight…then you do the dishes, and
head for the big comfy chair in the living room and collapse.
You are done for the night…but the morning is coming. And
my friend….again….this just the beginning.

Okay, Good Morning already yet. You arise at 4:00 a.m. to take
care of your loved one…before going to work… and if they
can't wash themselves because they are past that stage…then
"hello" it's up to you now. If they can do it for themselves, you
will have to do a few minor additions to the bathroom. If they
want to take a shower…fine, but you will now have to install
holding bars to assist them and bars on the wall and by the
toilet so they can hold on and satisfy their failing equilibrium.
Maybe purchase a seat riser for the toilet so they don't have to
sit down as far, and is easier to rise back up.

But if not, then you have the extreme honor of bathing your
loved one yourself. The beauty of all this is that you get a
chance to see what life is really all about and can be. So you
have bathed your loved one…and just when you are drying
them on the behind…THEY CRAP IN YOUR HANDS…
remember? Incontinence. So, you pick up your brains that
you have splattered all over the floor, and clean your loved one
again and yourself, and start all over. Now, throw away the
diaper and wash the clothes, and you're all set…are you? The
answer is a resounding "NO". This is just the beginning.

Chapter 5

I'm Going For A Walk, Somewhere

There are no stages in Alzheimer's disease. What may happen in the beginning can happen later on…and visa versa. You have heard of anger, walking, tantrums, etc, and the more you will hear, the more you will be able to deal with it all.

Let's take a nice sunny day during the week. So far up to now your loved one has managed to fend for themselves and you are still able to go to work. So, what may happen next is now the crux of what new decisions you are going to have to make.

During the day at some moment, you receive a call from the Police Department saying that they found your loved one walking aimlessly around the area, and would you please come and pick her up. Of course, this is going to make you leave work that day. Get ready if you don't already get the picture.

As you arrive at the station, you are greeted with the officiating officer who proceeds to fill you in, and then brings in your loved one….startled, your loved one asks the first question…. where am I?, how did I get here?". You reply …I don't know. And you don't.

Now some will have that problem early in the disease, some may have it during the time, and others may wait until later on to walk or not walk at all, and, if the latter be the case….you count your blessings. The danger here is that she could walk into traffic. Or hitchhike and lose her identity. Or worse yet,

they have been known to go to a bus station and take a bus…
and then where?

In my case, I was outside, just to show you that's how it can
ruin your day. I called to her inside and no answer…I looked
inside, searched inside…and checked the pool outside. I was
just ready to call the police when I went next door to my
neighbor's house and heard a "hello?"…In the front of the
house they had a little cove with a gate. Behind the gate were
the garbage cans…she had walked uneasily with her canes
to the gate, opened it, went inside, closed the gate, and fell
between the cans.

You see, at this point other things were happening. She started
having trouble with her foot. She had tendonitis in one foot and
could not walk very well. I got her a cane that my mother had
so she could use it now…had the operation on her foot, had a
boot for a time and was still not doing so well and went to two
canes…and she still walked there.

In Alzheimer's disease a person can almost will themselves
to do whatever they want to do if the mind is still able to
give directions. Now this is the only time she ever walked.
Others may do it over and over again…so let's say that is
what happens to you…now the question is, "WHAT DO I DO
NOW?" I might sound facetious, but, you pray.

Again the question comes up…."what am I going to do about
my job?" Again, the answer is, "PRAY BROTHER, PRAY"
You see now things are going to change radically and decisions
are going to have to be made quickly. What is the best

protection for you right now? You start putting chain locks at the top of each door to keep them from reaching up to unlock and open the door…now of course I am silly aren't I, you say, because you know they could get a chair and climb up on it and unlock the door…right ? Right! But it is doubtful that would happen however if that is a problem then you can purchase the kind with a padlock.

Now there is only one thing wrong with all this locking up business…You could be reported to the Department of Human Resources for elder abuse. WHAT…you say. Yes, that's correct. You have left that person incarcerated in their own home and that constitutes imprisonment and abuse. So, you ask again "WHAT DO I DO NOW?" Good question. Well, here are some suggestions, and you are the only one that has to answer the question for you are now an official caregiver…like it or not. And this is just the beginning.

Chapter 6

Total Care Facilities

Now, I know you want the best for your loved one and you want to take care of them the best way you can…you love them and you are responsible for their well being. Here are your choices. You can quit work and stay at home, never to leave your loved one alone, no matter where you go: to the post office, to the store, to an event, anywhere, you will take your loved one with you at all times, less you be reported for Senior Abuse. Okay that's step one, now step two. You can hire a day caregiver, at $25 an hour…now let's see, we mentioned that already…that adds up to big bucks. You are not Daddy Warbucks. (I just aged myself with that referral). They stay in your home from when you leave for work to when you get home. And the third option is…You will investigate a nursing home or assisted living facility.

First, let's look at the Assisted Living Facility. They are scrumptious and have all the amenities you would want for your loved one. There are a couple of types. One is a regular residence with 3 or 4 residents sharing a common kitchen, dining area, living room etc. Your loved one has their own bedroom with their own possessions, like a television for instance. It is not fenced or gated…that's not good if your loved one is "walking". In fact it's illegal for you to place them there, for they wouldn't accept them, had they known. Next is the assisted facility that has 4 or 5 residential houses that have 10 or more individuals living in their own apartments or large rooms. Again…if they are strolling off into the wild blue yonder, they may still be accepted. Here's why. The 1st residence is for those who can still work and drive. No problem, just a retiree with some failing health issue or just age alone. Then the 2nd house the same. The 3rd residence has a closer watch over all. There is a dining area in each place. A 24/7 nurse and or LVN, or CVN is provided for minor health needs. Some assisted living facilities are connected to a convalescent facility. But then the 4th and 5th houses come into play. The 4th is mildly restrictive, and has the same goodies as the rest. But the 4th is different. It is gated, and walled or fenced so that the resident cannot get out and start walking. They really don't know too much of what they are doing if they are to walk, but still can manage much of their affairs. And for those that are pretty well into the downward plunge, well, they are cared for as much as possible. They cannot get out. Now the cost? Hmmm, sorry about that. It will generally run from $1,500 for a 3-4 resident house to $6,500 a month for a class A facility with all the trimmings. That's $72,000 a year…can you hack that? Well, maybe you can and the glory of God be with you…but if you can not handle that, then there is the last choice - a nursing home facility. But wait, you can't just put them into the home without knowing if they will take Alzheimer's patients. And, that goes true for the Assisted Living ones also. One: the assisted facility may or may not have a nursing care unit attached to it. If it does, good. If it does not, that's not the place for you at this stage. And if they do not take Alzheimer residents…then you look elsewhere. "And where might that be?" you ask. Well, ask by phoning…

do they accept AD patients? And so now you have found a nursing home with AD care. Now what?

Hello, who is going to pay for it? A whole new change in your life is about to hit you square in your pocket book. So you ask yourself now…where is the money going to come from?!!!

The nursing home syndrome is not an easy task. Now you have no choice. The path is clear and you will have to place her in a nursing home. Now if you go to the county where the records are, you can ask for a list of nursing homes and their record of safety. But try to get one close to you.

Let's be reasonable for a second. You can't take care of your loved one the same way you did at home. Oh, I did comb her hair, makeup, trimmed and set her hair, make-up etc…I don't do it anymore, except once in a while. It is now in the hands of the nursing home. But, now you must figure on how to pay for it. This is what you will have to do. You will have to have her spend down anything that is your loved ones financial income or holdings. Down to no more than $2,270 in assets. (California) A car or the home does not count.

So, let's take a moment to evaluate. Assuming you have Medicare…but, let's not assume. What if you are not retired yet…oh a whole new picture and ball of wax. Now you have to depend on your 80/20 outdated health insurance plan. And it is not going to cover incarceration for a long period of time. You see you can't depend on your insurance to just continue. There will be a limit. Then you either have a good income or its time to apply for Med-I-Cal, and /or Med-I-Caid (California).

Then it takes about 4-6 weeks to get approved. And meanwhile the bill grows. Without an insurance plan that is going to assist you with this disease…you will see your financial world come down like a brick.

Now, let's discuss something briefly about your assets. First thing off the bat is that when you will find it necessary to place her in a nursing home or a special care facility, they will sometimes ask if you are receiving Social Security and request that you have their check signed over to the home. I recommend that you do not do this. The reason being, we know each other as a family and we do things for each other.

It is suggested that you get a hold of your attorney and have a Living Will and an Irrevocable Living Trust drawn up. This protects your estate from going through Probate which can be a costly procedure. The nursing facility cannot have it sent to them. Pensions also are not attachable. Have the check automatically sent to your bank. That's the safest way. Then you send your share of cost to the home. There may be other suggestions that the lawyer may bring to you.

Chapter 7

Protecting Your Loved One

What do I mean with the word "protecting"? Well, it's the extra little safety devices that you may or may not have to install in your home. You may not have to install them in the beginning because your loved one is still able to function well and is still coherent.

There may come a time, and it doesn't happen to everyone with AD, but to some it does and if it is your loved one that now is having trouble standing or walking or losing balance, this is now what may be suggested you do to prevent serious injury.

You may not see all of what is happening if you are away from the house and the loved one is alone, which I have already covered in previous chapters on that happening and your liability factors. But, if you are aware of what is going on and see your loved one fall, or is injured, or has other frailties that may hamper their daily activities, then you must, and I say, must do what is necessary at this stage.

Let's say, that your loved one takes a shower or uses the bathtub for their daily hygiene. Your loved one may begin to show instability in her walking now or her balance as I mentioned above, so you will need to install those safety bars in the shower and in the tub at lower levels that I suggested in a previous chapter, so that they can ingress and egress safely. Place them just as one would enter and higher also for the shower wall.

Then, what happens when they step out of the shower…you will need a bar for them to hold onto somewhere, or if need be their walker with the brakes on at the entrance. Make sure there is a non-slip bath rug to step on. And above all the towel racks should be close by to avoid over reaching and falling.

Now, the same goes for the commode. And, as mentioned before, you may need to add the riser seat so it will make it easier for them to sit and to rise from the toilet. A bar on the wall will aid that procedure.

Now, there is one more item. Lets say your loved one is doing fine except that they are a little unstable…and what if they fall and can't get up and you are not there…then they should have around their neck that "help" button that connects to you or someone to come help. The signal can be set to contact your alarm company or the fire or police department. My wife had one. She fell, lay there for sometime but didn't push the button because she didn't remember what it was for.

Is there more? Yes. What about just walking around? Maybe they are having trouble walking…and it will happen, because soon the motor skill will be attacked by the plaque. So then what…they need non-slip slippers or shoes. But that can be a danger too. My mother went to turn around for something and the non-slip did so well, she didn't move and went down to a broken thigh bone…so all things being equal…use your own thoughts on that.

Now it's possible they can't remember where to put the dishes if they are drying, and no dishwasher, or being on the blink. Then you find pots and pans in with the china. So you may have to label the cupboards where dishes, pots & pans, glasses, and the silverware are placed.

Another item of protections could be a chain around their neck that is attached to a name tag. It has their name and address on it just in case your loved one decides to take a stroll in the park. You may be able to purchase an identification kit at the local Alzheimer's chapter, or make your own.

The main thing here is to do what you have to do for your loved one to protect them the best you can. No, not all will have all these problems but you will have to deal with them one by one…and still hold on to your sanity.

Chapter 8

Personal Care When They Can't

The day has come now that you are going to have to bathe her, assist her in her toilet necessities. Why I say that is because you don't know what may happen to cause it. Wally had been having trouble with her right foot and was going to have to have it looked at for tendonitis. It went from bad to worse. She had to have a boot for 6 weeks. She had been a trouper when she accompanied me at events. Pain and all, she supported me and walked with me with the use of a couple canes. She started with one, then two, then the walker.

However she did her 6 week obligation and it was fine…until, she was still having trouble walking. Finally she had to have a walker. Now whether the plaque was destroying the cells related to her motorization I don't know but I do suspect that was what it was. However, she still had those necessary facts of life you do every day. But I could see now that it was going to be necessary for her to go to a wheelchair. One was ordered thru the private insurance company called SCAN, one of the leading plans available. And they provided one. Wally could not push the wheels because the ability to use and the strength of her hands was failing. The very thought of "how am I going to do this" came over me and I realized then that the road to nowhere would be a long one to follow.

The stress was mounting again in my weakened brain, and I was now feeling committed to doing what I had to do for her. This was the time that I really felt the strain and the extra burden placed on me. Washing her hair and setting it has been my forte for a long, long time. So I would manage to get her in front of the kitchen sink and put her arms on the sink to hold on to and let me do the honor of washing her hair. Sometimes she would come unattached and start to fall …but I caught her. Now the bathing…well, I gave her a sponge bath daily, and with that put on her first double set of diapers. I had figured out a way to do it.

Now you may have to sit down for this…I'll wait. As I washed her down at the kitchen sink I went to get her diaper on and ….that's right she did a bowel movement in my hand…great… and I guess I about flipped right then. So, I had to start all over again. She did it one more time getting her into the car. And I had to wash her all over again…I prayed for strength.

I could feel the frustration as the strength faded from me... but I pursued. I was diapering in the morning, noon, and at night I would put a double diaper on her. Oh, and by the way, you now have to wash their teeth, natural or false. And, what if the diaper doesn't hold and it leaks through to your bed mattress cover….I hope you have one. Well, then you have to get them up, clean them, get them in the chair, then clean all the rest and wash all the linen…you say you have to go to work and its 4 AM and you are tired ??? Forget it, you haven't seen anything yet. You love your loved one, there is no contention there, but you are beginning to feel aggravation because this whole thing is chipping away at your reserved strength and you are now very frustrated, stressed out, wanting to quit, your journal sounds like a mad person....and you are.

Taking care of someone who can manage for themselves under certain circumstances is one thing...having to do it under stress and aggravation is another and guess what...you are beginning to show the signs that I warned you about. Now what do you do?

If you are a spiritual person, then ask whoever you pray to, for help. Do what makes you feel comfortable. Then take a walk, but wait, you can't do that because that would leave your loved one alone....no, no, no, I say, you know you can't do that. Someone may see you and turn you in to the authorities...that is if you have a neighbor who doesn't care for you.

So, you don't go and your nerves are now on edge 24/7. Now is when you start thinking about the nursing home, before you end up in one yourself. AND THAT CAN HAPPEN. You can only do so much. And you will lay a guilt trip on yourself because you want to bring your loved one back to good health. Like I said before, you want information on her family history and genealogy. Find pictures of her family and label who they are if you don't know. Document everything. If they speak a foreign language, get all the important family history translated. Why you ask? Because in Alzheimer's patients, they may start losing their current tongue, lets say English, and revert back to their birth language. Now in my case it was the opposite. Because she was here so long, English was her natural language...and soon she could not read, write or speak her birth language. As I have mentioned before, I lost valuable time not getting some information down first before she lost her memory of those things.

The reason behind all this is that when they pass on, you will not be able to show your grandkids those pictures and tell them who they are or what it says in the inscriptions. By the way, they may not be able to write pretty soon, now what are you going to do?

Well you will now need to acquire 3 types of Power of Attorney. One for health factors, General, one for medications or other such as nursing home procedures, Special Power of Attorney and the third for signing legal documents and legal papers, Attorney in Fact. If you refinance…and you probably will…for this is going to dissolve what savings you have if you don't do this now…and you will be signing three times on each sheet of paper. You know how many signatures that is for 100 sheets of finance paperwork? Probably around 200 plus. One is her signature by you, the second is for your signature showing you have the POA and the third is for your own signature. It's a long time signing. I know because I have done it three times.

Now let's say they can't write or hold a pen …and you have to have something signed like the living trust I told you about. So now you have to get two witnesses and the Notary Public to verify. First you will try to help them sign if only an "X" then one witness that this is indeed their signature and the other to verify the mark was made and they also witnesses it. The Notary then carries out her duties. But from now on it will be you signing for your loved one…have fun…I did.

Oh there are still a couple of things you will be doing. Like going through the closets and giving away their clothes, because they will only need some for the nursing home if you have to put them there, and that's it. So, you will have to decide what to do with them - Salvation Army, friends, relatives or whoever may wish some of their clothes. So outside of a few things you will take over to the home, the rest will go, because they are not coming home again, at least on a permanent basis…for a visit, if allowed, yes, but that's it.

So, if you want to look at it from a more austere view, you are going to be alone in that big house, or apartment, and you are going to have to unload or pack away their belongings, just as you would if they had passed away. And, furthermore, you can say what you want, but you will soon after time you feel as if they had. For you are alone…kids, no kids, friends, no friends YOU ARE ALONE…so get a dog or cat… you will need one. You can play the hanging on syndrome, but you must face reality and the sooner you do, the saner you will be. Life offers no promises.

There is one other option here when you need help. There are many Home Care facilities and help that you can contract to receive help during the day when you may not be there or have to leave. Day Care is also available when you are not there or working. I have one here, for instance, named Angel Bear Adult Care. They come to your home and maybe take your loved one shopping or to the post office, or to have their hair cut etc. They will also do your laundry, change the linens, cooking, ….the things you may not be able to do yourself, or cannot take the time to do. You may find this service absolutely priceless in time of need.

Chapter 9

Answering To Your Family

Most likely you have children, grandchildren, or others in the family, young, or adult, that are going to be affected by the way you are acting or responding to your role as a caregiver.

Let's take your children. And let's say they are in their adolescent years. They now see you reviling from the stress of trying to make ends meet, taking care of your love one at home, and not knowing what is going to happen down the road. You have become irritated with the signs and actions of your loved one. Whether you are a mother, father, son or daughter, or relative in the role of caregiver, your personality is going to show changes to them. How do you explain to them what is going on?

First, write a journal as I have mentioned before, and write out your angers there for later when it's all over. You will refer to them and see for yourself the moments of despair. Explaining to the adolescents is heartbreaking because you have to relate to them in their language of understanding of what is happening and going to happen to the family and their world and how it will change. Oh, sure, kids go through having a loved one pass away and not being there any longer, but this is different. They are seeing the downward slide of the one they love and do not understand the significance or the definition.

The quiet, serene scene of their family life is now in flux.

They are observing special equipment being brought in, extra helpful maintenance and tools to assist the loved one in their daily routines. They see your personality changing every day… and usually it is with short tempers, irritability, impatience and withdrawal. If you don't sit them down and explain what is happening and how it may alter their lifestyle, because it will, they will be in total confusion and may withdraw themselves into their own cocoon. Ask for forgiveness and patience, for it will be a long ride through hills and dales and all must pull together, however, the one suffering ill effects the most, will be you.

Just speak with tranquility of the event and about the disease. An overall definition rather than the scientific breakdown for it will overpower them with medical mumbo jumbo. If they are old enough to understand, then explain the medical side of it, for by now you must have searched out the real definition and they can understand.

My daughter said…we are not the family as we were growing up, and we feel we have lost our mother, our father, and our former way of living and growing together as a family. She's right. You can't turn the clock back. What's done is done and you have to do what you have to do and deal with it as sensitively as you can. In a reality check, nothing remains the same and if you could alter the event, you would, but now you must keep the family as close as you can for you are going to need all the help and hugs, and kisses to give you support. Of course, if they do aid financially, that certainly will help. If they don't then it's all up to you to find a way to pay for it. If it isn't there, the tide will change and you will be caught up and sent out to sea…alone.

Let them become a part of the situation, if they are willing to of course, and to be the go between for this to be explained to their children. No one likes to see their loved ones fail in health or have those kinds of problems where there is no cure and no chance for it.

Is death kind? It could be. At nursing homes now, residents are often told they can pass on if the family doesn't come to visit, for the depression sets in and makes their stay harder for the staff. So, often it is whispered in their ears, "you can go now, you have lived a great life and although your family does not visit, you are loved" and literally, death has been known to take place not long thereafter.

Children are vulnerable to what they see. And to see something they don't understand is even harder. You must take the time to comfort them. Older siblings have a better chance of understanding the disease and accepting the end results, or at least knowing it will happen. They may not accept it. That's a problem they will have to live with and find resolution for themselves. If religious, then hold on to your beliefs, but be sensible and in a reality mode, for there is no cure and no turning back the clock. They are then forced to accept the fact that their loved one is leaving.

We are all children of God and we will all be together again. Now that's my belief, yours may be different and that's your belief. Just accept that the word "cure" is not the word of the day.

Be mindful of the anguish they are going through also and the effect on them to see you change and the hardness of your words. Try to be tolerant and know that they are suffering also. They need to have you for their strength as well. You have to keep your strength up and running. There will be quiet times, though few and far between. The grandchildren will be affected by their parent's reaction to all of this and they will need special guidance and knowledge about life and the events that are set in stone on what life can bring to the table and the answers on how to manage many decisions that will have to be made.

Visits are important and I can't emphasize that too much. If the loved one can still respond and have their faculties still intact to a point of self preservation, then children young and old will be uplifted spiritually and with forbearance of what is to be. And if the loved one does not respond anymore, then they need to be comforted and explained what is happening.

In time, as time marches on, they too will be at that point in life having to be cared for. That is not the future we had planned either, but life has its turning moments. The siblings have much to live for. Life isn't on a silver platter. For if one was raised that way, there will come a day when the balloon bursts and they will have to do with what they have. They too will see suffering and nursing homes and hospitals. But to take care of one at home requires more energy that one might express. Suffering is the key word here and it is here that it must be. You may not recognize the symptoms, but they do not. Don't be too concerned, young people have a built in mechanism to ward off imperfections.

Ten Warning Signs of Caregiver Stress

This is the crux of all that goes downhill when a caregiver begins the tell tail signs that he or she is having trouble coping with the monumental job of taking care of their loved one.

You must understand that you may be a raging maniac if you don't catch these problems and help to deal with them. Take a moment and read the warnings. I have been through them myself…I wrote letters and they sounded like I was losing my mind. I keep a journal to record my feelings all these years… it helps. And support groups are good if you are in to that sort of thing…many times I ended up giving them advice…its your thing to call.

1. DENIAL: Denying that the disease exists and its effects with the person who has been diagnosed. It is very natural to think that your loved one is going to get better…wrong. They won't…its terminal from the get-go. Some go early, some later…depending on the individual's body and its condition. So eventually you will have to let go. I know, you want everything to be like it was…won't happen, so get that out of your system right now. Why ruin your life at the same time…it can happen. Remember, you may die first just from the stress. That's a fact. The sooner you realize that you are heading for a train wreck and how to deal with the new life, the sooner you will accept it and move on with your life also. Learn about the disease. Get in touch with the association for further information and how it can aid in your recovery. Oh yes, you will need recovery from the stress of it all and its affect upon you. I know, I went thru the transition and as I look back…how fruitless it was to try and keep things as they were. It will take its toll and mostly on you for you cannot change what will be the end result for your loved one.

2. ANGER: Get ready, you are going to say things, do things, react to your loved one's condition in ways you never expected to do. Anger at them because they have asked the same question 10 times in an hour and you don't want to hear it again…but you must and you must answer quietly because they don't remember asking you the question. Like I did, record your anger in your journal. It will help down the line as you begin to accept the situation and be in the stage of reality. You may find that it is good for the soul to express yourself this way…you will need it. I piled it on my kids and that wasn't good for them…but they comforted me and gave me strength to carry on the best I could. And I did just that.

3. SOCIAL WITHDRAWAL: Well, that's up to you. If you are outgoing to begin with, you may just as well be with friends… and you will run into many people who have had a loved one with the same disease. And that's good for you to interact and talk. After all, they have been through it and all react in different ways. Some are rich enough to afford a 24 hour nurse. President Reagan had several on staff 24 hours. Nancy still suffered, but she didn't have to do the dirty work that the staff is there to do…It would have helped her I think. So, go out, meet others, and yes you could see periods of despair and not wanting to socialize. That's natural. But don't let it get to you. Force yourself to attend events…even after the loved one is in a nursing facility, you will need to because you are beginning to start your life anew, doing things as if you were single again. For me it was after 28 years of a loving marriage and respect and caring. You can't bring it back. You must not crawl into a shell.

4. ANXIETY: WOW, that is a big one. You will feel that emotion so much of the time because it is already over your head and you don't know what to do next…that's why this book…to help you with your emotions that are going to be thrown to the wind and scattered, and you wont be able to bring them together again until your loved ones passes on to a better life. But you MUST and I say MUST take care of yourself health wise. If you don't, you will suffer and fall prey to the demise I spoke of already. Take special herbs. Take Valerian Root to calm your system. Take Cayenne pepper capsules that will aid in absorbing the herbs. You don't need to add to the problem with the side affects of those drugs that are supposed to calm you down…the herbs will. I would strongly suggest that you not take Valium or other such downers because you can get "hooked" I know…years ago the Doctor ordered it for me…and after 30 milligrams a day and 10 years plus…I was… not a good scene…stay away from it. I am fully alternative medicine now and I do well. So, pamper yourself to relieve the pressure, it isn't over yet.

5. DEPRESSION: Oh boy. You will experience that without a doubt. To the point where you say…"I simply don't care anymore" but you see, you must. It's your health. You cannot do any more for the person you love. You are already extending yourself beyond the capacity to cope with the tragedy. That's why friends, going out with someone, having dinner with someone, attending concerts etc…will help you to maintain your dignity. You may feel like saying, "what's the use" but you must not quit. You must carry on and make those changes in your life to accommodate the need of the daily routines. After all, if you are still trying to care for them at home, you will need all your forces together to hang in there until the day comes to release that loved one to a caring facility. Listen to upbeat music, news, comedies. If you listen to the worse of the world events….it will bring you down with it. Pull yourself out of it…hopefully with your friends. If you feel you need someone to talk to and keep you company, have a real friend move in with you… that could help also.

6. EXHAUSTION: You are going to feel your strength begin to dwindle. That's why it is important that you take additional herbs and vitamins and good food choices to keep your strength up. If, let's say, in the afternoon, and you are going downhill fast, and without an ounce of get up and go, then take a tablespoon of honey and a tablespoon of apple cider vinegar mix and fill with 8 oz or more of water and guzzle…it will bring the potassium you need or take a banana which is high in potassium. I would suggest not taking drugs to do this…they will only wear off and make it worse. Get plenty of sleep if you can…8 hours plus…you will need it. Without it, you will feel the anxieties and frustrations more. Take your nap if you can in the afternoon. Now if you're at work and someone is watching over your loved one, then you can't, but your work will suffer because it is on your mind…and you are in the middle. Eat correct foods. There is strength there also…if you are a liver lover like I am…have it once in a while because of the vitamin A and energy it will give you. If you don't like liver…yeah, so what, you must keep your health in good shape. Stress can tear it away from you. If you feel sleepy or tired, and can hardly stay awake, then take the honey and vinegar, and, if you can, take a power nap for 20 minutes or so. Set the alarm.

7. SLEEPNESSNESS: Yes, it will happen. You will awaken during the night worrying, wondering, and trying to plan for tomorrow. And again, if you don't get proper sleep, you are not going to be able to handle it. It will rob you of your strength and ability to think straight for there is still much to do and many decisions to make on this road to hell. It's just beginning. Now if you take some calcium 1/2 hour before retiring, it will help calm your nerves and let you sleep, or Valerian Root (2 capsules). Take a walk around the house or outside if it need be…calm the system …warm milk and honey before will help also. And, you will say to yourself "I am too tired to do this" but you know what, you will have to do what you have to do.

8. IRRITABLILITY: Okay, so you are a grouch! Yep, its gonna happen. You will find yourself being negative in your responses to your loved one's questions or inability to do things for themselves. If you are a stay at home caregiver… it will manifest itself into you being a monster and not a nice person to be with, because what is happening is interfering with your life. You may even grow to dislike the person you are caring for. What you need to do, either in your daily routine of your job or just in your time of need, find other projects at home. Remember what I said about leaving your home to go to the store etc. and the liability it can cause you with the Department of Health Services, and they will charge you with elder abuse…so don't. If you can, take the person with you … if you can't …find someone to stay for a while. Again, dividing your interests up. If they can go with you to the store, all the better. You will get more and more irritable when they can't go with you and you have to make the other decisions. You may be more of a recluse, but let your friends know that you are and hold your hand out for comfort and friendship and love.

9. LACK OF CONCENTRATION: Let's see, where was I? What did I come into this room for? I forgot the appointment. I forgot to add this to the recipe. These are all normal. But it needs help so as not to become a habit forming reality. Do a little extra light reading. Watch a favorite TV show. Do a project to take your mind off your situation. Any activity to help you remain alert and able to administer to the needs of your loved one. Yes, you will feel that with your new responsibilities for the day, it will cloud your thinking process. Don't let it…you may forget or not even be aware….that your loved one has walked out the front door and gone somewhere. So stay alert for what may happen.

10. HEALTH PROBLEMS: Now this is going to be the focal point for you, YOUR health. Remember what I have been saying about that. You MUST take care of yourself. If you are not feeling well, have a health problem already that is being

affected by your new routines for the day, then take whatever
steps you feel you have to do to remedy the situation. If you
go to doctors…which I don't…thank God…and then go. Let
him fill you up with all kinds of pills and their side affects. Or
go natural and alternative to bolster your strength and needs.
Take Aloe Vera juice to help your daily needs in the nutrition
field. It contains all the natural vitamins, including the natural
vitamin B-12, amino acids, and enzymes that your body needs.
You can't afford to get sick…your loved one needs you to
help them. But if you don't get help from whatever source you
choose, you could start the downslide of your own demise…
and it has, and it could, and it will happen if you don't take care
of yourself first.

There are going to be financial worries also but this too will be
managed. Think positive for the night is young and it isn't over
with yet.

Chapter 11

The Nursing Home Visit

You are not in charge of her care anymore, so get over it.

I say that because you are NOT in charge anymore. Once you have gone through all the paper work, let alone the Med-I-Cal paper work which will take about 4-6 weeks before you hear…and then they may ask you to present them with more information. I had one year a reply back that asked me about a deposit in our account for $17.25…you will feel that you have just been audited. But that is how they will begin to undress you, down to your toes. So, get used to it, you will have to re-approve them every year. It does get easier because the original information doesn't change very much.

Okay, now your loved one has been admitted. They are smiling at you, and even talking at this particular stage, and even moving…so you ask yourself, then why did I have to put her here?. I could have continued to have taken care of them at home. NO, YOU COULD NOT!! That's why you are sitting in the office signing more papers to put them there because it had reached that point of either being them or you that would be going into the nursing home.

Now look, if you are well healed and bundles of dollar bills lying around, you may wish a more appealing atmosphere and desire a nice Assisted Living Facility. Yes, they are nice. A beautiful dining room, music, waiters with white gloves, some I saw with their mink jackets on attending their nightly meal.

But believe me you will pay for all that service. You can have a sleeping room, a one bedroom, a two bedroom and a suite if you like, it's your money. And that's wonderful IF you can afford it. But at $6000 plus a month times twelve comes up to $72,000 a year. And if you think you can handle that with the $500,000 you have in the bank, think again. That will be gone in 6.9 years…and then you are broke, and end up still being in a nursing home with Med-I-Cal assistance on the financing, so why didn't you go there in the first place and still have the sanity and the funds to take care of yourself? Maybe your share of the cost will only be $550-1000 a month…get the point? Good. You may have more to say in an Assisted Living Facility, but that may be mute because your loved one is on a downward slide and may soon be a vegetable laying there staring at you, and you can't communicate anymore. Do you still want to pay $6000 a month - for what? The nursing home is medically staffed and your loved one can still stare at you, not talk, and be a vegetable there as well as in an expensive assisted living facility.

What I am trying to get across to you, is that it is time for you to give them up to those whose job now is to take care of your loved one the best they can. Will there be mistakes? Yes, and I have lived them, but let me tell you about the facility you will visit everyday.

Get to know them personally. I am like a member of the staffing family and I enjoy the camaraderie that begins to envelope you. I play the piano at special events there or just for lunch or dinner sometimes. It makes them happy to hear older songs. I comfort those residents there and help them when I can.

The facility like a nursing home is not a private entity owned by a big organization …some may be. The nursing home is usually in a group of several homes under their direction. So the umbrella corporation in charge has just one thought in mind…..MONEY!! And they will make changes in the home if necessary to make sure they are getting their slice of the pie. You see, the wing that makes the money is the one that is one day in, and out in only a few days or a couple weeks, or the private rooms, which bring in the bigger bucks.

Need insurance? Yes you will supply that and along with Social Security if you are retired, and/or Med-I-Care or Med-I-Cal. Now, some insurance says you will pay for ambulance service if your loved one needs to be transferred to a hospital. However, if just on Med-I-Cal assistance, they will pay for it. That could save you $150 right there. So I cancelled my insurance for her so that she would be covered if that be the case. Besides she had run out of all the days she could have for a year when entering. So choose wisely.

Now, let's say you are visiting. And, they can manage for themselves until one day they cannot. The hands may not grab the fork. So you can go and help her and feed her or let the staff do the task. As it is, the whole country is short of CNN's, CNA's, LVN's, and nurses. Some come from out of the country and there is a language barrier sometimes. And of course you want your loved one taken care of just like you did at home…

FORGET IT, it aint gonna happen. They will provide what is necessary according to the Health Services Commission in your state that governs nursing homes and facilities. Some of the Assisted Living ones have a small urgent care unit attached. They generally insist on your loved one being able to walk and take care of themselves. Once the resident can not…then they may ask you to transfer her to one having less expensive and have more accommodating arrangements.

There is a note of warning for you though. If you think you are going to go into a nursing home and because your loved one did not have a light bulb replaced over their bed or any other little concern, and you make a big stink about it and other minor things every time something happens…hear this: The nursing home HAS THE RIGHT to ask you to not visit anymore, for you are causing an upheaval in the daily operations and upsetting the other residents, or to just transfer your loved one to another facility. Do you get what I am saying to you? Why bitch and bitch and bitch…and then have to transfer them…and start all over again with the paper work and the aggravation only to find that the next nursing home has the same minor infractions. And you did this for nothing.

Now, if it was a major infraction or problem…yes that can happen. And then you take it to the first line of authority, the director on the floor and shift nursing staff. Then she will take it to the Director of Nursing and the Director of Nursing will take it to the Administrator. If you think you are going to call in the militia, think twice. You may be hurting yourself if you indeed transfer to the next nursing home that will be aware that

you sued the last one or called in the Health Services unit…
and they may not take you. So where does that place you? The
best is to go through the chain of command. Discuss how the
incident happened and what can be done to correct it. They will
work with you and possibly terminate individuals if necessary.
In any case, work with the home and they will work with you,
don't make it any harder or more stressful for yourself. If there
is abuse, that can be dealt with immediately and with evidence
and the same termination can apply and that person will never
get another job in that capacity…and you have had your day
in court. Work with them whenever possible, you are just
making it more difficult for your loved one and less attention
to their need may occur without your knowledge, and you
can't be there every minute. Simple things can be corrected
like leaving trash on the floor, dirty linen, etc, etc. can be
peacefully corrected, and they will be thankful for your input
and concern. C'mon, they don't want an unannounced visit by
the Health Services or the Board of Health either…they will
work with you and for your loved one. You can make yourself
heard, just no need to shout, in the long run it doesn't pay, and
you will still have to put them in some facility. Now like I said
previously, lets say you can afford the first 6.9 years…then
what when the money runs out….and your loved one with this
debilitating disease may live another 10 years. That's what you
have to consider. The money will run out if you are not really
financially capable to handle it. And you will have to downsize
everything. Maybe even sell your house or move to a cheaper
apartment. Remember what I said…YOU MUST TAKE CARE
OF YOURSELF. So do it!

There is one last resort if all else fails. This is done
occasionally depending on the circumstances, and that is...
you divorce your loved one. I know, no one can answer that
but you. It's done for several reasons. One, to be able to afford
their stay in a facility if you can't in any way do so. The other
is to reduce your responsibility for financial support if the
money isn't there, from a legal standpoint according to the laws
of your state. I have seen it happen, but it wasn't for me...I
couldn't do that. But it happens.

That's why care giving is so much more stressful than if the
loved one had passed away, and all you had to do is make
arrangements, which you will have to anyway, and not feel the
burden of the loving responsibility that will soon engulf you
and bring pain and stress into your life. If you like that then go
for it...but you may end up in the box sooner.

Yes, I am being rather crude...why not...life is crude
sometimes and if you don't realize it yet...then that's why I
am writing this book - to warn you and give you some criteria
for surviving yourself. Scare you? You bet, for you are going
to change ...in your attitude toward others that you love...it
will show up and they will say ...gee I'm sorry. It's not pity
you want, its undying love of others and the caring that others
who have been through this can give to you, and a shoulder on
which to rest your weary head.

There is another subject which you will have to consider.
You must think of it now. The average number of years that
an Alzheimer's disease victim may live is about 8 years. The
average stay, and that is "average' in a nursing home is 2.5

years. But I know of many going past that statistic. However, let's say your loved one does manage to continue to live for some time. But the day or night will come when you receive a phone call, saying that your loved once has passed away. Now what do you do? If you have made the proper arrangements then there won't be the question usually asked. But, if you have not then here is what will be asked. "Mr. Smith, where do you wish for us to send your wife (or husband if Mrs.) Do you have a pre-paid funeral plan? Have you ever given any thought to who, what, where, and when of that audacious moment in time? So be prepared to give an answer. Go out now and purchase a pre-paid plan for you and your loved one. The average cost of a funeral these days are around $7000. I won't go into all the ramifications of the whole process, I was in the funeral and cemetery business for years and that is something you will need to do ASAP.

Now, let's say for a scenario, in the middle of the night, you receive a call that your loved one refuses to eat and won't open their mouth. And they have discussed it with the doctor who has ordered the insertion of tubes to feed her. Is that what you want…a bunch of tubes sticking in them?

Okay, let's go on, one night you get a call that the organs are failing and the doctor has ordered a life support system be attached to your loved one to keep them breathing, even though the brain is dead.

Still, going on. One night you receive a call that your loved one had a heart attack 30 minutes ago. The CNN just discovered it on her visit to her. The first thing is the resuscitation and immediately the Nurse on duty will carry out CPR along with the pounding on the chest to try to re-start the heart. Then after determining that they have expired, the Paramedics are called. When upon arrival they put your loved one on a flat board and AGAIN pound the chest with force to try and start the heart. And only after it is realized that the person has died, do they then make the official pronouncement.

Now my question to you is…DO YOU WANT YOUR LOVED ONE TO GO THROUGH ALL THAT PHYSICAL ABUSE? I should hope not. And for what? To continue living in a shell, a vegetable, and where there is no life to sustain in their condition? No, I didn't want that either. Let them go. Let them be without pain and suffering, let them be where they will not be ravaged with this disease and return to our Maker.

So, now you know what you wish to do to avoid the automatic procedure that will take place when there are no written instructions otherwise. Well, there is. Go to the admittance representative and sign the papers that spell out your wishes against: 1. tube feeding, 2. life support systems and 3. resuscitation.

And then, if that event occurs on either front, it is clearly stated and they will not attempt further procedures. You should do that upon their admittance to the facility. You never know, and whether any of us do, the time, the place of our leaving this realm of iniquity. Yes, you will have to make that decision to stop feeding them if they refuse to open their mouth for anyone, and have sealed their lips so you can't invade the stronghold. The muscles of the throat have ceased to function and they can not swallow, which is called "aspirating". Then this must be a family decision if that be the case…to order that the person be taken off the feeding schedule, conditional upon the fact that the person refuses to cooperate and has continued for 3 days to resist the food. Then the body will begin its normal shutdown. The liver and the kidneys will go first. The last organ with be the heart muscle.

This is hard to contemplate, but absolutely necessary. It may be the hardest decision you will have to make, but make it you will - for them and for your sanity.

Chapter 12

Now I Am Alone
Let Go – Let God

It is done. Your loved one is now in an assisted living facility or a nursing home, and you now go home to an empty house… oh sure….maybe the dog greets you at your door. You now enter and you are feeling completely exhausted for you have spent valuable time taking care of your loved one, and not getting much sleep. There's all the equipment, wheel chair, walker, portable potty, tons of diapers, clothes, personal affects, pictures, medical equipment, maybe a special bed, canes, all the equipment that you needed to make your way through the day to do what you had to do to try and keep your sanity and yet take care of your loved one.

The air smells of alcohol rub and medicine. Next the aroma of your loved one's after shave lotion, her perfume, the hair brushes…all the reminders as if your loved one has passed on…God, what a horrible state of mind you are now in. You may think you are alone… but not really. There is a feeling of relief that will pass over you first. For now, your life is now ready for you to take over and move on. You must think of yourself now. If you don't, you will be in such a facility yourself.

You are now….the survivor….yes that is what you are, your loved one may not have passed on but you are now left to fend for yourself. You will cook, if you haven't already, you will clean house, if you haven't already, in other words, life is now up to you.

Maybe the loved one is a parent. This is a situation which can affect your life is you are married…or single. IT WILL TAKE MUCH OF YOUR TIME. You will feel lovingly obligated but it will change your life as you now know it.

Why? Because you will be spending time, not only in visiting but in preparing the documents every year if you're on a government program such as Medicare or Med-I-Cal. But that person will be on your mind. I am not so concerned about families who are affluent being able to afford the $6000 a month for Assisted Living Facilities if that is where that person is residing. They have wonderful facilities and nursing care if needed. The fact that it is not like a nursing home, they have their own apartment and needs. If they still are walking, they will do fine. BUT, If your loved one cannot do these things, or has just been diagnosed with AD, then you will want to make sure everything is going ok…refer to Chapter 6.

You have accepted who, what, where, when, and how. Now you must make certain decisions. What if you have children? A facility takes money. If your loved one qualifies, then you will have to pay a share of the cost depending on your combined income. Remember in Chapter 6, I mentioned that your house and auto do not count. But their assets at this writing can only be $2270. Okay, I know you're asking. "Well what about if we have more as their assets?" Then of course as I mentioned, you will be spending down…yep…you have to get rid of her holdings so that it is no more than the amount above. That's how it is in California, check your state's regulations. Now for yours, if you are working, have your own business etc., this all plays into the final amount. If you are thinking of re-financing your home to help pay for all this, not fret, that's a loan, not income, on your mortgage. However, don't sell yourself short. Cases like President Reagan's, can last for 15 years or more. The average stay in a nursing home is 2½ years. But with AD it can be more because maybe the mind is gone but the body lives on and if you don't cover it up front, then you may have to re-finance again down the line.

Now what about the clothes and other effects? Well, you will have to see that your loved one is clothed at the facility with their favorite outfits …sometimes it wont be much because they may be bedridden and wont need as much. You will mark with a permanent marker and then list all their clothes to the facility. They will sew in a permanent label with their names. Will clothes get lost? You bet! But make sure there are sufficient quantities. Please, Please……DO NOT TAKE EXPENSIVE JEWELRY. Some costume is okay, but some costume jewelry can be expensive. Yeah, I know, you are asking…"You mean there is theft in those places?"….You bet there is and you wont be there to see it stolen, so get use to it…I remember one resident lost her false teeth….never found…probably thrown out in the bed sheets. Pictures, some memorabilia is fine, depending on where the person is. Oh, what about hair? Well, there is generally a beauty shop on the premises. But you will be filled in with all that. But that's a bit of the time I am talking about, that you will be spending seeing that your loved one is being taken care to the best of your best ability…but remember what I said in chapter 6.

What about the rest of their clothes, considering they are not returning home and are pretty well cemented to the facility and not expected to leave, then you will have no other alternative than to give them away. You must start making that void in the home that is going to happen and fill it with positive statements. Fill it with joy, and happiness, and the family. If no family, have friends over, anything to stem off the loneliness. Now know this, no one can feel what you have been through but you. They have their own cross to bear.

If you find it is still too much, change the furniture, whatever, to move on with your life…why? Because if you don't, you will be mired in your loneliness and it could be so devastating that you could cross through the vale yourself, even before your loved one…as I said in the beginning, **65% OF CAREGIVERS DIE BEFORE THEIR LOVED ONE!!** (That's a proven statistic.) Now, you must take control.

You're Alone? No, your family is there, your loved ones, your friends that love you and support you and don't forget…GOD is there with you…you must now let go and let GOD help you, for you are his child, he will give you strength. And, when the day comes that your loved one has moved on to a better place and without the disease, you will feel that all is well, and you have done all you could, and taken the right steps to enhance your life for as many years as it was, or will be, necessary. That is where you also will need the patience.

You will still make the visits and see that all is well and if they need anything. Like I said before, you are no longer in charge, the facility is, and you must work with the facility to make it happen. Let them know you stand by to help in anyway to make your loved ones life comfortable.

Alzheimer's disease, Parkinson's, Lou Gehrig's disease, and other spinal deformities, are in need of stem cell research. Make yourself known and your opinions on that subject…It is my own belief, you are not killing a baby, because they are not breathing yet…when a breath occurs, then there is life, and what's left over would have been thrown out with the bath water.

You are lucky if your loved one can speak to you, love you, kiss you, hold your hand, and comfort you. Unfortunately, in my situation, she is immobile, unable to speak, move or even feed herself. You might say a vegetable, but to the children, they are still there for them…and you, if there is any subconscious working, but you may not know that. But to the kids, they still believe there is communication. Be glad for them, but soon they too, must accept the fact of reality. If you don't, you will not let go.

Then when you have started a "new" life…without your loved one, you will have to make decisions without her and on your own. Eat out alone? Never?…well, you will. Life goes on whether you are here or not, so if you are going to be here, you might as well live it the best you can and move on in life. Here, comes the hard decision. Your loved one has been there and now may be in a debilitated vegetable state and you know that this is not the life for them or you. If you are Christian then you know you will both be together again, but if you are not, then you still may worship in your own belief system and ask for your loved one's comfort for you don't want your loved one to suffer anymore than they have to…but its time now to have to say goodbye to your loved one. Therefore, you and others do preach to the one God. Now you do the same…and ask God to take your loved one. Don't feel as a caregiver, you can not hold on forever. Remember what I said earlier. God will act in his own time…I just don't want you to feel that you put a guilt trip on yourself.

You have supported your loved one for years already. Let them go to be without the disease. Also, pray that we get a cure for all of them. Then after you have released your loved one, you must whisper in their ears, "you can leave now." They are waiting for you to say that they can go. Do it. It took me a long time to mull that over in my mind. And once I did, I was free of any possible guilt. Sure, at the funeral you will feel the obvious sadness, but remember…THEY ARE NOT LOST, for you know where they are. Easy? No, it's not, but nursing homes have been doing that for years.

The road of life is filled with potholes, curves, and low hanging branches. You must carry on through all of the pitfalls. Learn from them; give creditability to that which has been proven correct. You have the will and the authority to speak for yourself and let others know that you have let go, and you have let GOD into your corner, and if you are not of a faith based belief then search for guidance or support that will provide you with the strength you will need. As one spoke in times past giving me strength to endure for my own needs - "Tough times never last, tough people do."

E N D

Bibliography

Alzheimer's Association Progress and Report
5900 Wilshire Blvd., Suite 1100
Los Angeles, California 90036-5036

Dr. Noreen A. Bumby, D.O.
Gero-Psychiatrist, Clinical Investigator
Studies results with Southwest Clinical Research
71-511 Highway 111, Rancho Mirage, California, 92270

Personnel Testament
Thirteen years with on hand experiences

Internet applications and search on Alzheimer's disease

Discussions with other caregivers and their experiences.

Research into Med-I-Cal (California) and Medicare
requirements

Lawrence Adler, M.D. (original diagnosis)
Desert Medical Group
275 N. El Cielo, Palm Springs, California 92262

Nursing Home operations and policies
Premier Convalescent and Rehabilitation Center
2990 East Ramon Rd
Palm Springs, California 92262

www.ingramcontent.com/pod-product-compliance
Lightning Source LLC
Chambersburg PA
CBHW031259280526
45784CB00004B/1916